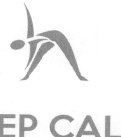

KEEP CALM
AND GET FIT

Keep Calm and Get Fit:
150 Bodyweight Exercises
You Can Do At Home
For The Perfect Total Body Workout

By: Little Pearl

CONTENTS

YOUR HOME, YOUR HEALTH, YOUR BODY

Any successful person will tell you that in order to get what you're after you need to have an amazing reason for why you want it. You can't just set the goal of wanting a million dollars – you'll never get there if the number is all you think about. Instead, you have to think about what that million dollars will do for you. How will it change your life? What will it feel like when you have it? What is the real, emotionally charged reason for wanting it? This type of thinking is the only way to actually get what you're after.

Staying fit, losing weight, getting in shape – all of these goals are no different than saying you want a million dollars. They are vague and, by themselves, not motivating. You might be thinking right now, "Hang on, I do want to lose weight!" Or, "Yes my main goal for working out is getting in shape! What's wrong with that?" But these types of vague goals only touch the surface of a deeper desire – and leaving your goals like this make it incredibly easy for your mind to find a way out.

Your mind is the most powerful tool you have when it comes to training, which is why your first step towards getting fit needs to be convincing your mind so that when your body gets tired and the sessions get long, your mind won't give you a way out. It will push you, keep you going, and, in return, get you the results you have been wanting.

So before you even begin working out, ask yourself really why you are doing it. What will it mean to you when you hit your goal? How will you feel? What will you get out of it? Picture all of this in your mind and feel as if you have already attained it. Show your mind right now that it is possible. Tell yourself that no matter how tired you are or how much you would rather be doing something else, it is all worth it because of the satisfaction you will have of actually attaining your goal.

Remind yourself that your body is more than just skin and muscles and bones – it is your home. Your body is always with you, reminding you of the decisions, whether bad or good, you have made. And based on those decisions, your body is determining your current health. How you are eating, breathing, thinking, and working out are all affecting your present state.

You have the ability to change all of this.

You can make a better home and a better life for yourself. You have all the tools you need right now, right where you are. The question is, will you?

WHY BODYWEIGHT TRAINING IS THE MOST EFFECTIVE WAY TO WORKOUT

Bodyweight training is the key to creating effective, no-excuse workout routines. Unlike overpriced, over-marketed machines and equipment that tend to isolate only major muscle groups, bodyweight training works every muscle of your body, including key muscles that keep your body safe and healthy. Many of the top fitness trainers in the world are switching from equipment-based workouts to bodyweight workouts and here's why:

- Bodyweight exercises require your body to **cultivate balance and stability**, which means you are working more muscles and keeping your body safe.
- Bodyweight exercises **can be done anywhere** – no excuses like gyms being too expensive, too far, or that you were traveling. Plus, you can workout outside!

- The variety of bodyweight exercises **keeps workouts fun and challenging**, which means you won't quit or dread your workouts.
- Bodyweight exercises are **accessible to everyone** – men and women of all fitness levels will see results.
- Bodyweight exercises **improve range of motion**, which allows you to perform daily activities more safely, effectively, and comfortably without risk of injury.
- Workouts that rely on bodyweight exercises are **more efficient than other routines** because you can work several muscle groups at once while simultaneously working your cardiovascular system. This means that you don't have to spend as much time working out and the results will be even better.
- Bodyweight training **increases your metabolism** faster than other forms of exercise, which means unwanted pounds and fat will disappear more quickly.
- Because balance and stability are essential in nearly every bodyweight exercise, **the core is constantly being worked**, which means faster results with fewer repetitions of core-targeted workouts.
- Bodyweight exercises don't just **build muscle**; they **improve your flexibility and your stability** as well. This means your body won't just be something nice to look at – it will work better too.
- It's easy to **do bodyweight exercises with a friend or a group**. This is a great way to keep yourself accountable, to have fun, and to have someone there to push you when you start to get tired or want to quit.
- **Bodyweight exercises actually work!** Research shows that the results you will get from this type of program are far better than any other.

WORKOUT STYLES AND PLANS
FOR EVERY BODY

Your workout style depends a lot on your personality, your goals, and the amount of time you have to dedicate. All of the following styles are effective so long as you do them correctly and at full intensity (you get out what you put in). It's best to alternate between the styles on various days – this leads to faster results and it's more fun.

- **Interval Training:** The basic premise of interval training is to increase your heart rate as quickly as possible by alternating between exercises with minimal, if any, rest in between. Usually the exercises done in one interval vary in degree of difficulty, meaning you would include one or two really tough exercises with ones that aren't quite as demanding. For example, you could do 1 set of 3 different exercises in a row, and then repeat it 2 or 3 more times so that you get 3 sets of 3 different exercises total. One of the benefits of interval training is that it allows you to work to your maximum effort without burning out a specific muscle group all at once – your arms could have time to rest after a set while you do a set of leg and core exercises. Other perks of training with intervals is that you tend to burn more calories and improve your cardiovascular fitness, which means you will be able to run, walk, climb, whatever, longer and faster.

- **Ladders:** Unlike interval training where you switch between various exercises, ladders vary the number of reps that are done in one set. For example, you could do your first set of exercises with 15 reps, the second set with 20, and the last with 30. Traditionally you then work your way back down the ladder, repeating the sets of 20 and 15 in this example. Ladders are a great way to target a specific area and are ideal if you work out with a friend since one person can do a set of reps while the other person rests and so on. Short and efficient, ladders are a fun way to train.

- **Time Trials:** This style of training let's you get the most out of the time you have to spend, even if it's just five minutes. Choose the exercises you want to do, grab a stopwatch, set a goal time, and go! See how many reps you can do, maybe even write it down, and then try to beat yourself next time. Fun and speedy – there are no excuses!

- **Power Yoga:** If you have never done Power Yoga you're in for a surprise if you think yoga is easy. Power Yoga is comprised of sequences of difficult bodyweight exercises that challenge your balance, strength, and endurance. It provides a nice alternative for those days when you get sick of counting reps or are feeling like a bit of stretching intermingled with your workout would be a good idea. In addition to toning muscles and building strength, this workout style teaches you to be aware of your breathing and provides an effective way for managing stress too.

THE PLANS

1. **Lose Fat:** In order to lose fat you need to stimulate fat-burning hormones when you workout. According to experts, to trigger these hormones each set of exercises you do should have between 10 and 15 reps in order to be most effective. Additionally you should aim to do at least 25 reps total of an exercise, which means at least 2 sets. So your workout plan should look something like this:

   - 3 Sets of 12 Reps of 5 Exercises: 1 Arms Exercise, 2 Legs Exercises, 1 Core Exercise, and 1 Full Body Exercise.
   - Do this workout 5 times each week, choosing different exercises each time.
   - In addition to your bodyweight exercise, you should aim to get 20 to 30 minutes of cardio exercise every day, like walking, jogging, hiking, or swimming.
   - After 4 weeks, increase the reps and sets – you will be looking so good and strong too!

2. **Build Muscle:** Building muscle requires causing damage to the muscles through strenuous exercise. Most of the time you think of damage as bad but it isn't the case here. The acute trauma that muscles receive when you workout forces the body to repair the muscles and when they do so the muscles become thicker and larger due to the influx of satellite cells that have come to the rescue. Because of this damage and the necessity for your body to repair, it is important to allow muscle groups to rest by alternating which exercises you do,

focusing on different areas each time you workout. Here's an idea of what an ideal workout would look like:

- Monday – 4 Arm Exercises, 2 Core Exercises, 1 Full Body
- Tuesday – 4 Leg Exercises, 1 Core Exercise, 2 Full Body
- Wednesday – Rest
- Thursday – 3 Arm Exercises, 3 Core Exercises, 1 Full Body
- Friday – 3 Leg Exercises, 1 Core Exercise, 3 Full Body
- Saturday – 1 Arm Exercise, 1 Core Exercise, 1 Leg Exercise, 3 Full Body
- Sunday – Rest
- Aim To Do 3 Sets of 8 – 10 Reps of each exercise

NO EQUIPMENT, BODYWEIGHT EXERCISES

Before you get started, it's important to keep a few things in mind to make sure you get the most from your workout while avoiding injury.

First, proper form is always more important than number of reps – it's more effective (and safer) to do fewer reps that are done well than to do more that are sloppy.

Second, fast isn't always better. Try doing some of your reps slow, taking your time moving through the motions rather than rushing and see the difference in how your muscles work.

Lastly, always keep in mind that you get out what you put in. These exercises require you to give maximum effort in order to get results – don't cheat yourself by holding anything back!

> *Note: Some exercises require you to hold still or to do as many as possible for a specific time, so rather than do reps follow the time indicated with each specific exercise – this counts as one set.

Arms

1. Push Up

   * Place your hands and feet just wider than shoulder width apart, body in a straight line with the ground. Look just ahead, not down, and squeeze your butt and your abs. Arms start out straight and so do the legs.
   * Bend your elbows and lower down as much as possible. Do your best to keep your elbows from sticking way out to the sides as you lower.
   * Once you have gotten as low as possible, pause, and then straighten the arms quickly to come back to the starting position.

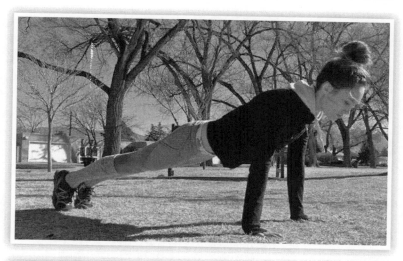

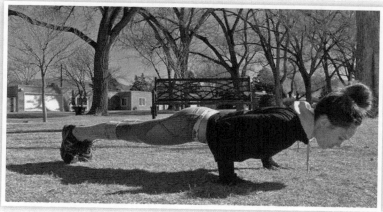

2. Diamond Push Ups

- These are done with the exact same method as the regular Push Up only with fingers touching under the body so that the index fingers and thumbs form a diamond.
- This type of push up works the triceps more than the regular version.

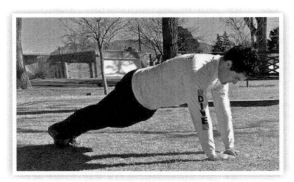

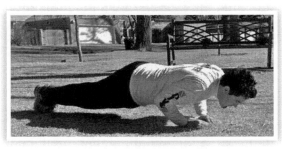

3. Extra Wide Push Ups

- These are done with the exact same method as the regular Push Up only with hands out wider than shoulder-width apart.
- This type of push up is more difficult than the regular version because you have less leverage to push yourself up.

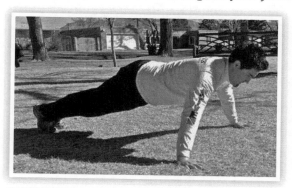

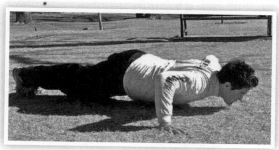

4. Triceps Dips

- You will need something like a chair (bench or stairs work great too) to do this exercise.
- Place your hands on the chair surface, fingers pointing towards you.
- Straighten your legs out in front.
- Keep your elbows in line with your shoulders as you bend them to lower down. Pause and press your arms straight to come back to the starting position.

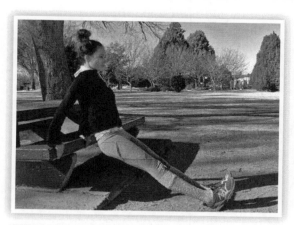

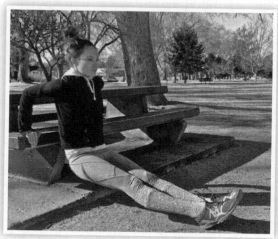

5. One Leg Dips

- These are done with the exact same method as regular Triceps Dips only one leg is lifted to increase the weight your arms bear.

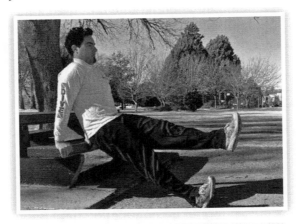

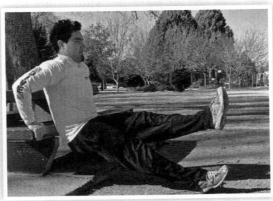

6. Reverse Triceps Push Ups

- Start lying down on your stomach with your hands under your elbows.
- Come on to the balls of your feet and lift the knees off of the ground.
- Engage your core and press your body up just high enough so that your elbows are in line with your shoulders. Be sure to keep your body parallel, not allowing the butt to get too high or low.

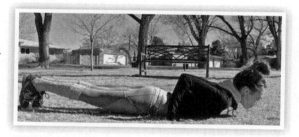

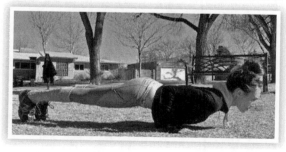

7. Alligator Push Ups

- Starting at the top of a push up position, bring your knee to the outside of your arm.
- With the foot lifted off the ground, complete a regular push up.
- Switch legs for the next rep.

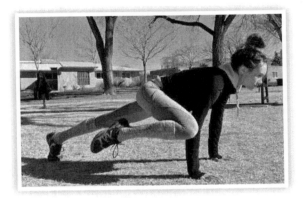

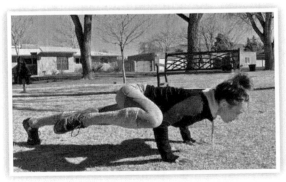

8. Staggered Push Ups

- These are done with the exact same method as the regular Push Up only with one hand 6 to 8 inches further in front than the other.
- Unevenly distributing your weight makes the lower arm work harder than the arm that's in front.
- Alternate the arm in front for the next rep.

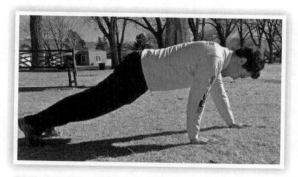

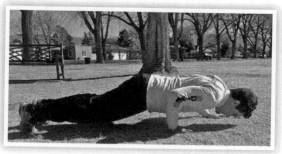

9. Bi-Level Push Ups

- These are done with the exact same method as the regular Push Up only one arm is bent with your weight on the forearm instead of the hand.

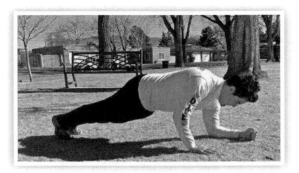

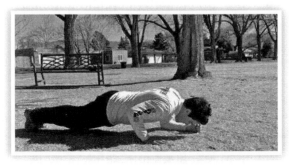

10. One Leg Push

- These are done with the exact same method as the regular Push Up only one leg is lifted off of the ground.
- Keep the lifted leg straight with toes pointed down.

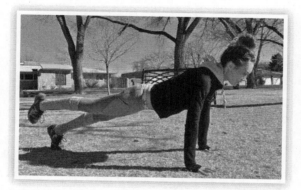

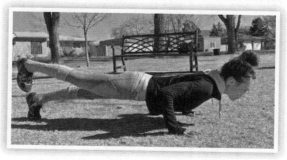

11. Handstand Push Ups

- Come into a handstand position (unless you're a super g use a wall).
- Bend the elbows just as you would in a regular pushup, making sure they don't come out too far to the sides.
- Pause at the bottom of the push up before straightening the arms back into a full handstand.

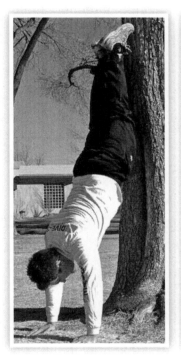
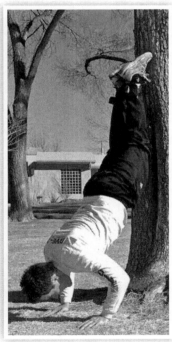

12. Wall Walks

- Kick your legs up a wall, just above a 90-degree angle. You should be facing away from the wall.
- Start with your hands under your shoulders.
- Walk your hands away from you as far out as possible without moving your feet. Pause and then walk your hands back under your shoulders.

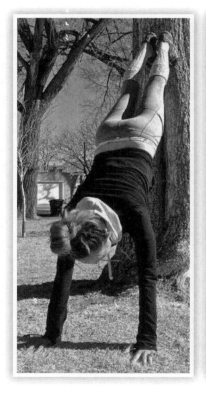
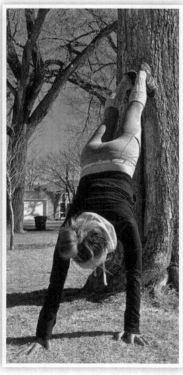

13. Incline Push Ups

- You will need something like a bench, chair, or stairwell for this exercise.
- Come into a push up position with your hands on the elevated surface. Perform a push up as you regularly would.
- This version targets you shoulders more than your pectorals and is easier than the standard push up.

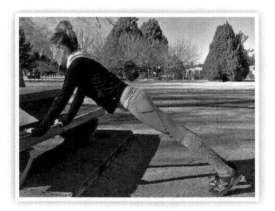

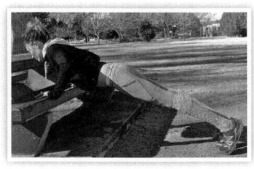

14. Decline Push Ups

- You will need something like a bench, chair or stairwell for this exercise.
- Come into a push up position with your feet on the elevated surface. Perform a push up as you regularly would.
- This style of push up puts more pressure on your wrists than the regular version. To help keep your wrists safe, walk your hands forward a bit more than usual and turn them out slightly.

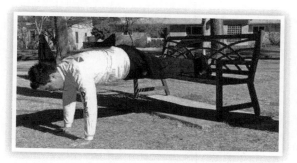

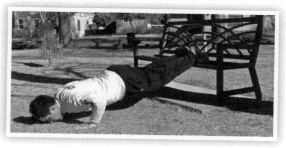

15. Single Leg Decline Push Ups

- These are done with the exact same method as the regular Decline Push Up only one leg is lifted.
- Alternate legs between reps.

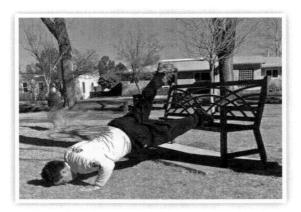

16. Crossed Reverse Push Ups

- Sit down and bring your hands behind you, slightly further than directly under your shoulders.
- With legs straight, cross one ankle over the other. Lift your hips off of the ground.
- From straight arms, bend your elbows but keep your hips from touching the ground. Press arms straight to come back to the starting position.
- Switch legs between reps.

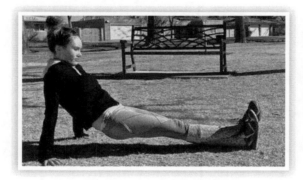

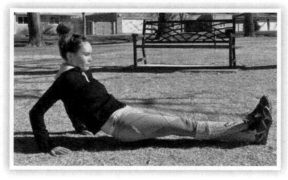

17. One Hand Push Ups

- These are done with the exact same method as the regular Push Up only one hand is placed behind the back.
- These are really difficult, which is why there is no real demonstration-- Good Luck! *(If by chance you are a one-hand push up master, send us an email – support@littlepearlpublishing.com - with a photo and the first person will be featured in this book!)*

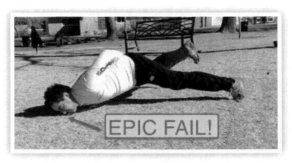

18. Clap Push Ups

- These are done with the exact same method as the regular Push Up only a clap under the body is added.
- Rather than come back up to the top of the push up with straight arms, after you clap drop straight back into the bottom of the push up with bent arms.
- In order to have time to clap, you must press up from the bottom of the push up more explosively. This, of course, takes more strenght

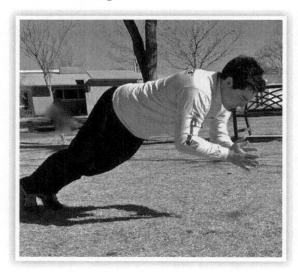

19. Dolphin

- Come to all fours with your forearms on the ground. Place the palms of your hands flat on the ground, directly in line with your elbows.
- Lift your knees and straighten your legs.
- Look forward slightly as you walk your feet in as close as you can towards your elbows. Once you have come as far as you can, hold this position.
- Aim to hold for 45 seconds or as long as you can – this is one set.

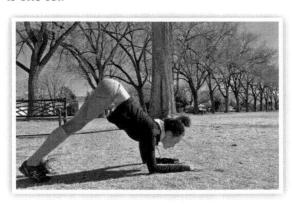

20. Forearm Hold (Forearm Hold)

- If you have never done this before (or even if you have), use a wall to help with your balance.
- Kneel down facing the wall. Lower your forearms to the ground, hands 3 to 5 inches away from the wall.
- Your palms should be flat and directly in line with your elbows.
- Straighten your legs, keeping the forearms down, and begin to walk your feet as close as you can towards your elbows. You now look like you are in Dolphin.
- Look forward and kick your feet up towards the wall, just like you are coming into a handstand.
- Hold this position for 30 – 45 seconds – this is one set.

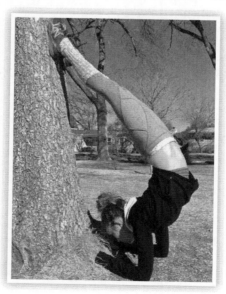

21. T Push Ups

- These are done with the exact same method as the regular Push Up only after pressing back up to straight arms, open to the side balancing on one hand and the side of the foot.
- Alternate sides after each rep.

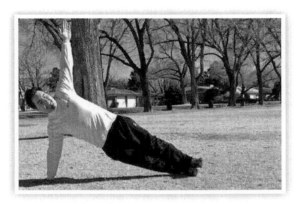

22. Chaturanga Push Ups

- Start at the top of a regular push up.
- Walk your hands back a few inches from under your shoulders. Keep them right next to your body.
- Bend the elbows to lower down, but keep them in contact with your ribs.
- Pause once you have lowered to the point that your elbows and shoulders are in one straight line (hands should be under your elbows).
- Straighten the arms to come back to the starting position.

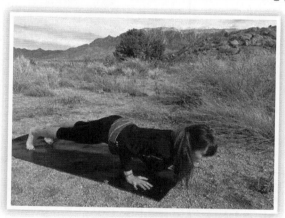

23. Down Dog Push Ups

- Start on all fours with straight legs, hands just in front of the shoulders, hips lifted.
- Bend the arms and lower just as you would in a regular push up, keeping the hips high.
- Straighten the arms to come back to the starting position.

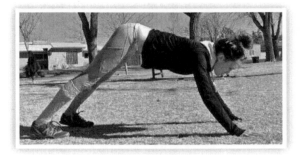

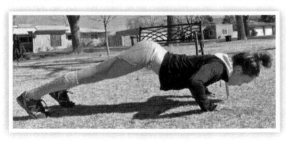

Legs

1. Sumo Squats

- Stand with your legs about 2 feet apart, toes pointing straight forward.
- Keeping your weight in your heels, bend your knees as if you were going to sit in a chair behind you.
- Keep your back as straight as possible.
- Straighten the legs to come back to your starting position.

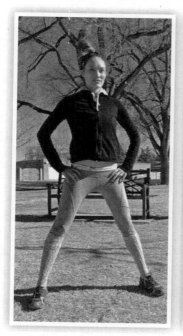 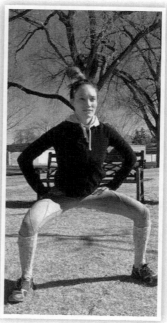

2. Crossed Lateral Lunge with Extension

- Stand with your feet a little wider than hip width apart.
- Bend one leg and step the other foot behind you as wide as possible. Get as low as you can while keeping the back straight.
- Straighten the front leg as you come back up, swinging your back leg out to the side and as high as you can.
- Come back to stand and repeat on the other side – this is one rep.

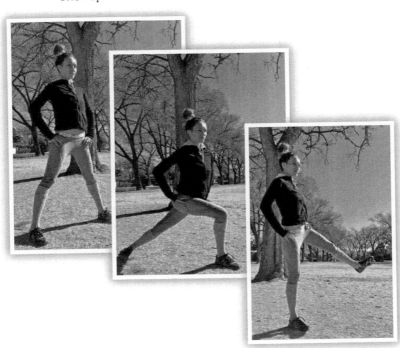

3. Elevated Foot Lunge

- You will need a chair or a bench for this exercise.
- Stand 2 to 3 feet in front of the elevated surface. Place one foot on top of the surface.
- Bend your front leg to lower into a lunge – make sure your knee does not come out further than your ankle. If it does, step further away from your back foot.
- Straighten the leg to come back to your starting position.
- Do all of your reps on one side before switching legs.

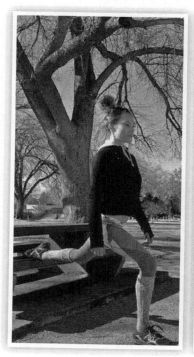
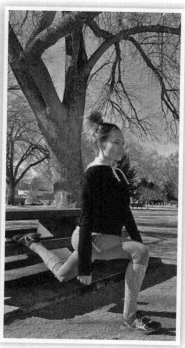

4. Squat Hops

- Stand with your legs just wider than hip width apart, toes pointing straight forward.
- Bend your knees to squat doing your best to keep the back straight.
- Sink down a little lower in your squat and then explode into jump. Land back in the squat – this is one rep.

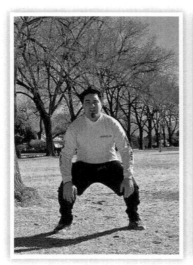 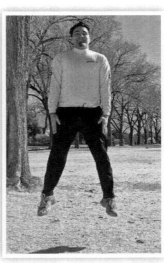

5. Lifted Heel Sumo

- Stand with your legs about 3 feet apart, toes pointing out slightly.
- Bend your knees and lower into a deep squat with knees to the sides and ankles directly beneath.
- Lift one heel off of the ground, pause, and then lower the heel back down. Repeat with the other foot for one full rep.

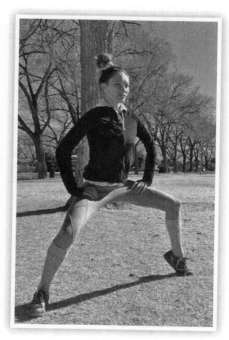

6. Double Lifted Sumo

- This exercise is done exactly like the Lifted Heel Sumo (link to "Lifted Heel Sumo") only both heels are lifted at the same time instead of just lifting one.

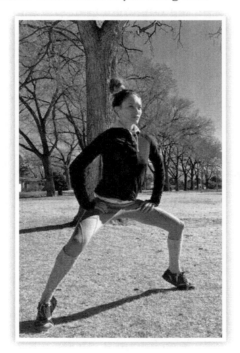

7. Box Jumps

- You will need a sturdy surface, such as a chair or a bench, to do this exercise.
- Stand in front of the elevated surface with feet together.
- Bend your knees and jump up, keeping feet together and knees bent.
- Hop back down to finish the rep.

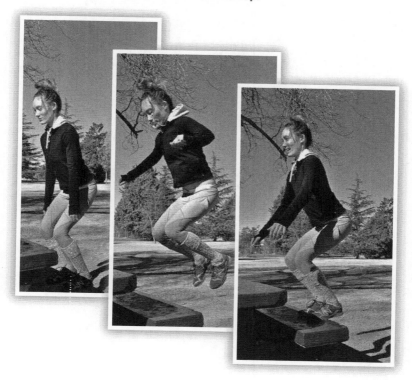

8. One Leg Box Jumps

- This exercise is done just like regular Box Jumps (link to "Box Jumps"), only you jump with one leg instead of two to increase difficulty.

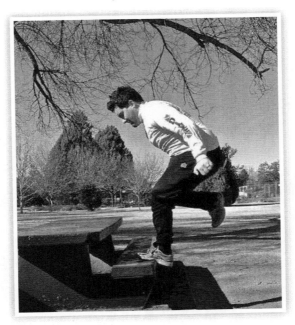

9. One Leg Squat With Kick

- Do a low squat with knees together, keeping your back straight and weight in the heels.
- Shift your weight into one foot and lift the other off the ground. Pause here.
- Kick your lifted foot out in front and straighten the leg as much as possible, while keeping your other leg bent in a semi-squat.
- Come back to your starting position and repeat with the other leg for a full rep.

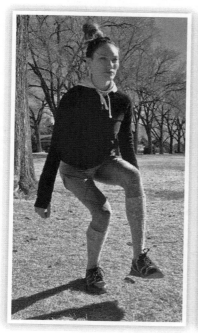 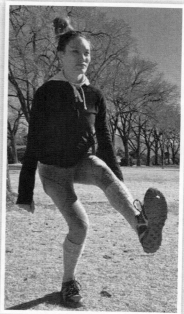

10.   Lateral Leg Lift

- Lie on your side with legs stacked on top of each other.
- Flex the feet and lift the top leg straight up as high as possible.
- Lower the leg slowly down to the starting position.
- Do all of your reps on one side before switching legs for a full set.

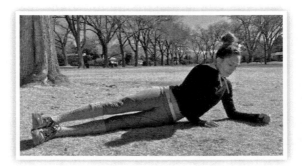

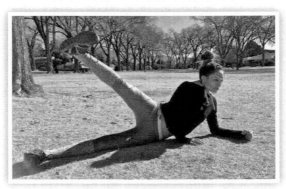

11. Lateral Leg Circles (Lateral Circles)

- This exercise is done just like the Lateral Leg Lift (link to "Lateral Leg Lift") only the reps are completed by circling the top leg rather than lowering and lifting.
- One full circle is one rep.
- Do all of your reps on one side before switching legs.

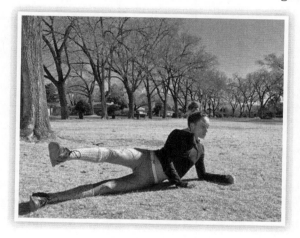

12. Lateral Leg Pulses

- The set up for this exercise is just like the Lateral Leg Lift.
- Once the top leg is lifted, lift the bottom leg off of the floor.
- Pulse the bottom leg up and down – these count as your reps.

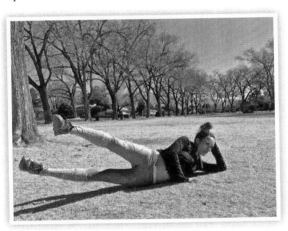

13. Hop Switch Lunge

- Take a big step forward with one foot, setting up for a regular lunge.
- Bend your front knee, keeping it directly over the ankle and lower your back knee down towards the ground.
- Explode into a jump on the way up and switch legs, landing into a lunge. This is one rep.

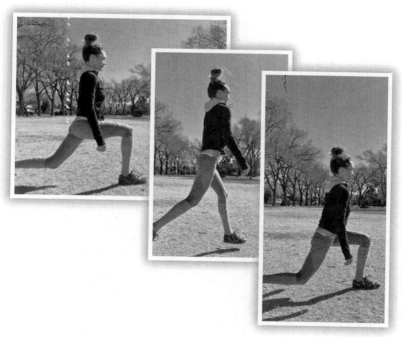

14. Elevated Bridge Lifts

- Lie on your back with your feet on an elevated surface, such as a bench or chair. Feet are hip width apart.
- Press your feet into the surface and lift your hips off of the ground.
- Be sure to keep your head still when doing this exercise.
- Lower the hips back down to the ground to finish one rep.

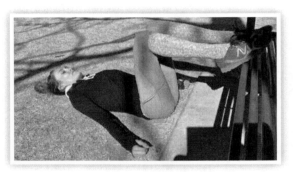

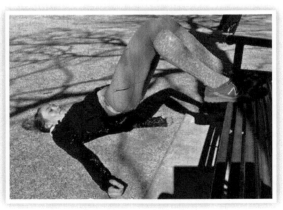

15. One Leg Elevated Bridge Lifts

- This pose is done just like the Elevated Bridge Lifts except one foot is extended up into the air to increase intensity.

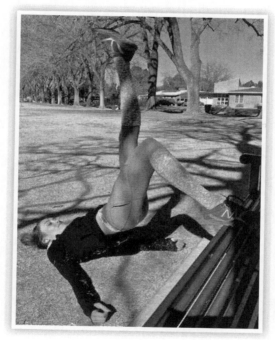

16. Jumping Butt Kicks

- Stand with your feet together.
- Bend your knees as if you were sitting into a chair.
- Explode into a jump, kicking your butt before your land back into the squat. This is one rep.

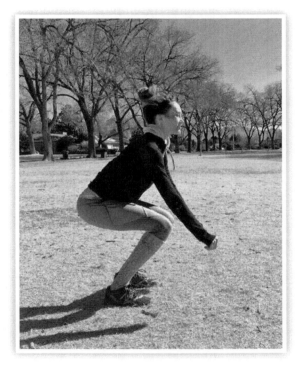

17. Pistol Squats

- Stand with your feet together. Lift one foot off of the ground.
- Keep the lifted leg straight as you bend your other knee into a squat. Get as low as you can before coming back to stand.
- Don't let your lifted foot touch the ground at any point between reps if you can help it.
- If it is too much to do all reps on the same leg at once, alternate legs after each.

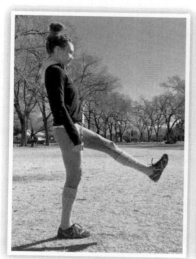
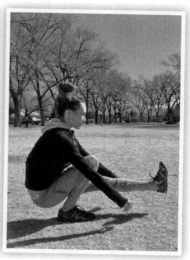

18. Lunge Kicks

- Take a big step forward with one foot, setting up for a regular lunge.
- Bend the front knee to come into a lunge.
- Shift your weight into your front leg and swing your back leg forward. Straighten your front leg as you do so.
- Bring the lifted leg back and return to a lunge to complete one rep.

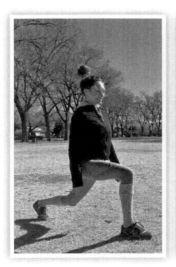 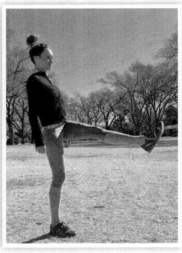

19. Single Leg Bridge Lifts (SLB Lifts 1 and 2)

- Lie flat on your back with knees bent and hip width apart. Place your feet directly under your knees.
- Lift one foot off of the ground, extending the leg straight in front of you as parallel to the ground as possible.
- Lift the hips off of the ground as high as you can, pausing at the top before lowering the hips back towards the ground.
- Repeat all of the reps on one side before switching legs.

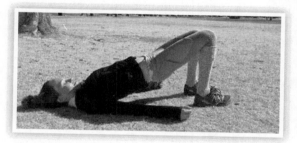

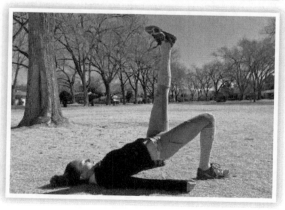

20. Calf Raises

- Stand with your feet together.
- Lift onto the balls of your feet and pause at the top before slowly lowering the heels back down to the ground.

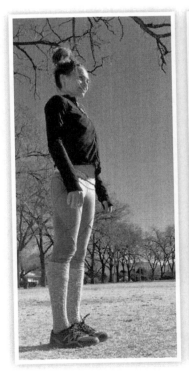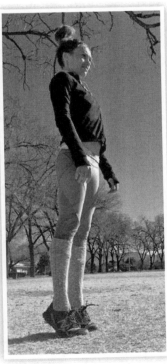

21. One Leg Calf Raises

- Lift one foot off of the ground and bring it to the back of your other leg's calf.
- Lift onto the ball of the foot and pause at the top before lowering the heel back down.
- Do all reps on one side before switching legs.

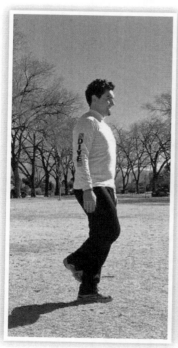
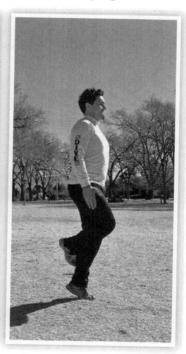

22. On The Edge Calf Raises

- You will need to stand on the edge of something to do this exercise – a stair or curb is perfect.
- Stand on the edge of the elevated surface so that your heels hang off lower than your toes.
- Lift into a calf raise slowly and pause before lowering the heels back below the toes.
- Doing calf raises on the edge of a surface gives you a bigger range of motion, which makes this exercise more difficult and more effective.

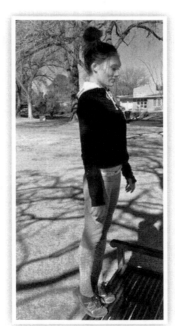

23. Teapot Tips

- Stand with your feet 2 to 3 feet apart.
- Keeping the back straight, bend your knees and squat. Be sure to keep your knees behind or right above your ankles as you do this.
- Shift your weight into one leg, straightening it as you lift the other leg off of the ground.
- Reach your hand down to the ground and lift your back leg so that it is parallel with the ground.
- Slowly lower the lifted leg and come back to a wide squat.
- Repeat this exercise on the other side – this is one rep.

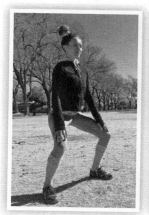
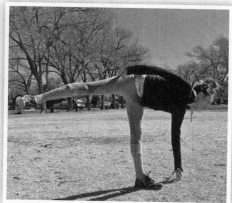

24. Standing Lateral Leg Raise

- Stand tall with your feet together.
- Shift the weight into one leg as you lift the other leg to the side as high as possible without moving the hips.
- Lower the leg back down to starting position.
- Do all of the reps on one side before switching legs.

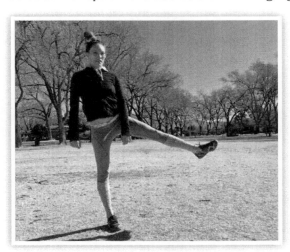

25. First Position Squats

- Stand tall with your heels touching and toes pointing out.
- Keeping your feet in this position, bend the knees and come into a squat.
- Straighten the legs to come back to the starting position.

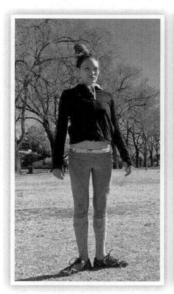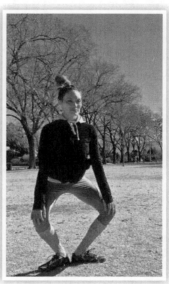

26.   Third Position Squats

- Stand tall with one foot in front of the other, the heel of one foot touching the arch of the other.
- Keeping your feet in this position, bend the knees and come into a squat.
- Straighten the legs to come back to the starting position.

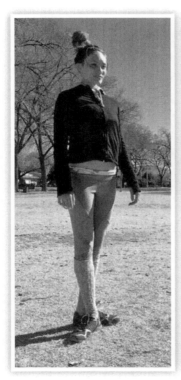 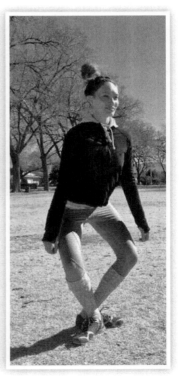

27. Back Leg Lift

- Stand as tall as possible with your feet together.
- Keeping the back straight and without leaning forward, lift one of your legs back as high as possible.
- Return the lifted leg to the ground but just lightly tap the toes between reps (don't come all the way back to stand).
- Do all reps on one leg before switching.

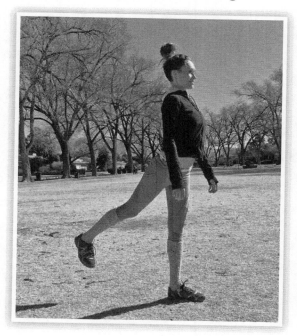

28. Bent Back Leg Lift

- Stand as tall as possible and lift one foot off of the ground. Spin the inner thigh forward and the knee to the side.
- Standing tall, lift the leg back behind you as high as possible, keeping the inner thigh facing forward.
- Lower the leg back down in between reps but don't allow the foot to touch the ground.

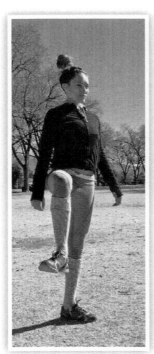
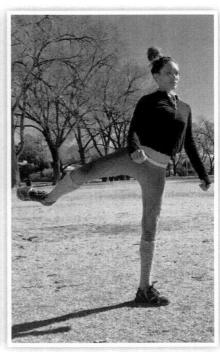

29. Donkey Back Leg Lift

- Stand as tall as possible with your feet together.
- Keeping the back straight and without leaning forward, lift one of your legs back as high as possible.
- Bend the knee of the lifted leg and try to kick your butt.
- Straighten the back leg but keep it lifted. Pause before going to your next rep.

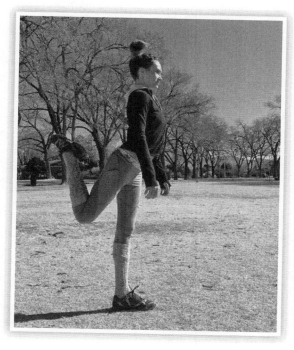

30. Front Leg Raise

- Stand tall with your feet together.
- Shift your weight into one leg and point the toe of the other foot. Lift the foot as high as you can, keeping the leg straight.
- Lower the foot back down to the ground, just lightly tapping the toe, before moving onto the next rep.
- Do all of the reps with one leg first and then switch legs.

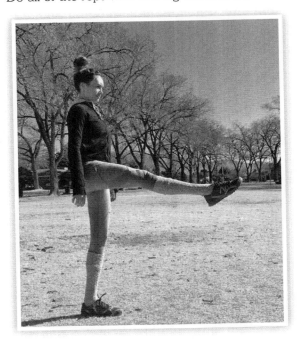

31. Step Up Back Leg Lift

- You will need a sturdy elevated surface, like a bench or chair, to do this exercise.
- Stand in front of the bench facing it.
- Use one leg to step up onto the bench. Straighten the leg you stepped with as you lift the other leg as high as possible behind your body.
- Keep the foot that has stepped onto the bench in the same spot in between reps so that you can move more quickly with less rest.

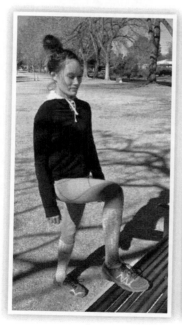 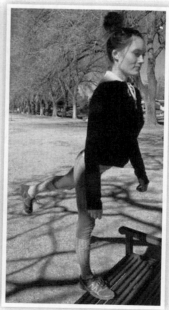

32. Step Up Side Leg Lift

- This exercise is done just like the Step Up Back Leg Lift only instead of extending the leg back you extend it to the side.

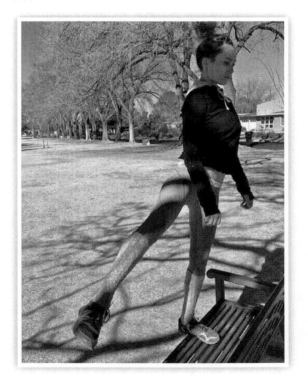

33. Step Up Knee Hug (Step Up Hug)

- This exercise is done just like the Step Up Back Leg Lift (Link to "Step Up Back Leg Lift") only the lifted leg is brought forward and the knee is hugged into the chest.

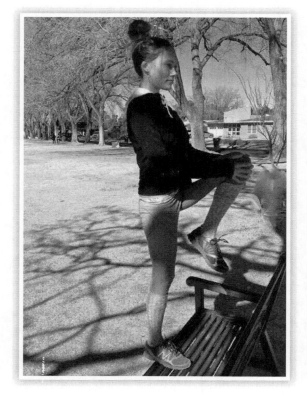

34. Lateral Step Up

- You will need a sturdy elevated surface, like a bench or chair, to do this exercise.
- Stand next to the bench.
- Use one leg to step up onto the bench. Straighten the leg you stepped with while lifting the other leg out to the side.
- Lower the extended leg back to the ground and step off of the bench – this is one rep.

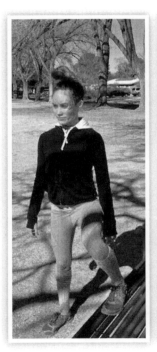
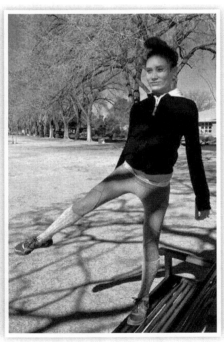

35. Front And Back Circle Hops

- If you have something handy to make two circles on the ground (like a hose, dog leashes, etc.) go ahead and do so, placing the circles about 3 feet apart. If you don't do this just imagine there are two circles and don't cheat yourself!
- Stand in the center of one circle with feet together facing the other circle.
- Bend the knees for power and, keeping the legs together, hop forward into the second circle.
- Land with bent knees and immediately hop backwards into the circle you started in. This is one rep.

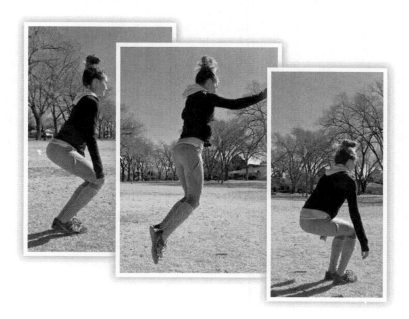

36. Lateral Circle Hops

- This exercise is done just like the Front And Back Circle Hops only instead of jumping forward and back you jump side to side.

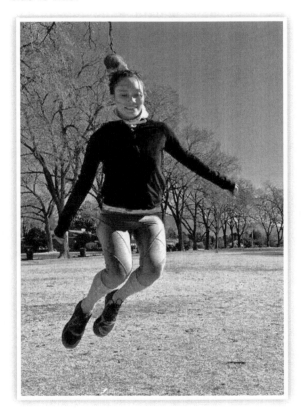

37. Squat Calf Raises

- Stand with your feet together.
- Bend the knees and imagine sitting back into a chair be-hind you.
- Keeping the knees over the ankles, lift onto the balls of your feet and pause before lowering the heels back down.
- Stay in the squat in between reps.

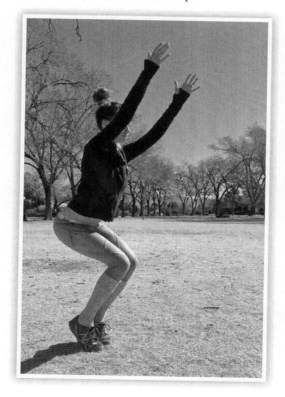

38. Super Low Sumo Stand

- Come into the lowest squat possible with legs as wide as necessary to get the heels on the ground. Turn your feet out to the sides to protect the knees.
- Reach your arms over your head and straighten your legs to stand, keeping the arms over your head.
- Bend the knees and come back down into your super low squat – this is one rep.

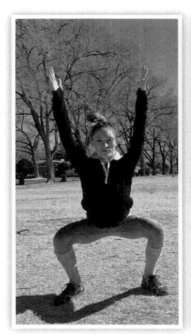 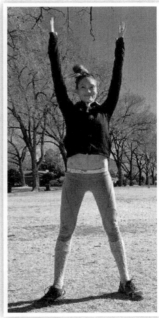

39. Dancing Monkey

- Step your feet 3 to 4 feet apart.
- Bend one knee to lower your body down towards the ground and straighten your other leg out to the side.
- Without using your hands, shift your weight so that you extend your bent leg and bend your straight leg, switching sides. This is one rep.

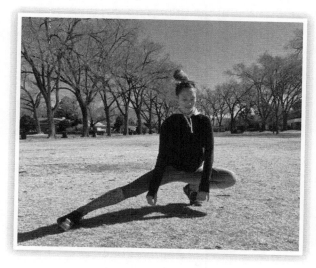

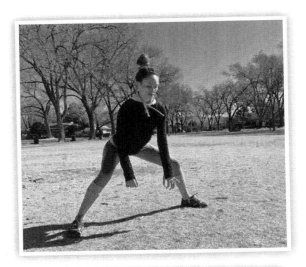

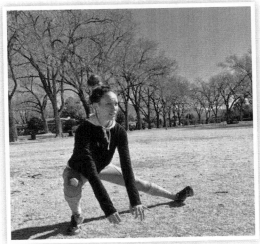

40. Hands Down Squat (Hands Down)

- Stand with your feet together and legs straight. Bring your hands to the ground. If your hands don't touch with straight legs, find something to place them on like a low step.
- Keeping your hands on the ground, bend your knees and squat. Be sure your knees stay over the ankles and not in front.
- Keep your hands down as you straighten the legs again to finish the rep.

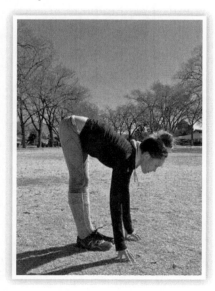

41. Lunge Lifts

- Take a big step forward with one foot, setting up as you would for a regular lunge.
- Bring your back knee down close to the ground as you bend your front knee.
- Start to straighten your front leg as you lift your back leg up, balancing on one leg, body parallel to the ground. Reach the arms forward and pause before slowly lowering back into your starting lunge.
- Complete all of your reps on one side before switching legs.

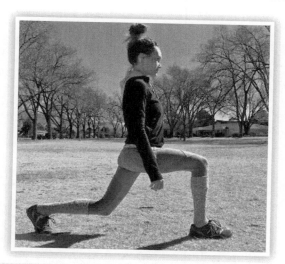

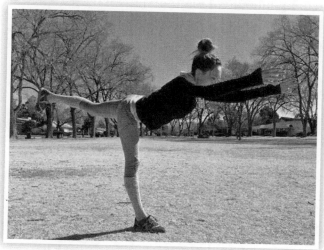

42. Fire Hydrant

- Come onto all fours.
- Lift one knee off of the ground and to the side.
- Lift the leg up as high as possible, keeping the knee bent.
- Hold this position at the top for a moment and then slowly lower the knee back down, not allowing the knee to touch the ground between reps.
- Do all of the reps with one leg before switching.

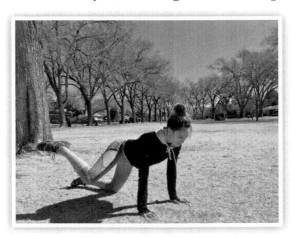

Core

1. Boat

- Sit on the ground and rock your weight back so that you balance on your sit bones.
- With bent knees, lift the feet and the hands off of the ground.
- Keeping the back straight and the chest lifted, straighten the legs.
- Continue to lift the legs as high as possible for as long as you can, trying for 30 seconds – this is one set.

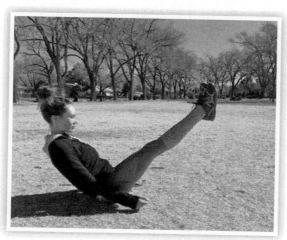

2. Paddle Boat (Paddle)

* This pose is done just like Boat only the legs flutter rapidly up and down as you hold for the 30 seconds.

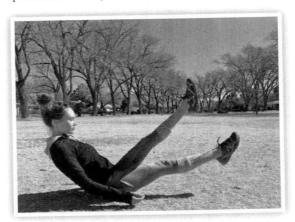

3. V Sit Ups

- This pose starts out just like Boat.
- Once in Boat with legs fully extended, lower your upper body and your legs down towards the ground. Hover just a few inches away from the ground and then return to the Boat position.

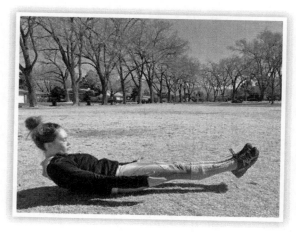

4. V Crunches

- This pose starts out just like Boat.
- Once in Boat with legs fully extended, bend the knees and bring them in towards your chest. Pause here and then extend your legs back out to the full Boat position. This is one rep.

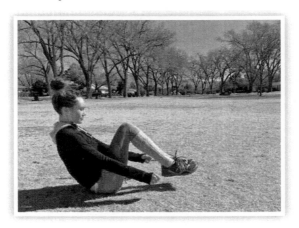

5. Center Split Crunches

- Lie flat on your back with legs extended straight up into the air (perpendicular to the floor) and arms reaching over your head.
- Lower one leg down towards the ground, hovering just an inch or two from actually touching. Keep both legs straight.
- Lift your shoulder blades off of the ground as you curl your body up towards the lifted leg, hands on either side but not touching.
- Lower very slowly back to the ground, keeping the legs just as they are.
- Do all reps with one leg before switching sides.

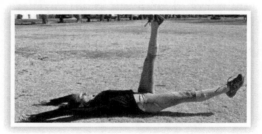

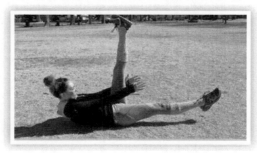

6. Side Split Crunches

- This exercise is done just like Center Split Crunches only the arms reach to the outside of the lifted leg, adding a twist to the crunch.

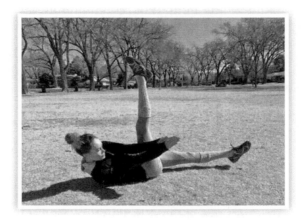

7. Plank

- Come onto your forearms, legs extended straight out behind you.
- Press your forearms into the ground and lift your body so that it makes one straight line, parallel with the ground.
- Do not let the hips get too high or too low in this position.
- Look forward slightly to keep the back of the neck long.
- Try to hold this position for 45 seconds or as long as you can – this is one set.

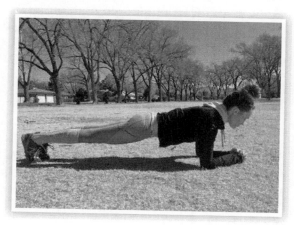

8. Plank Taps

- This exercise is done just like Plank except rather than just holding for 45 seconds, lift off of one of the forearms and tap the palm of the hand to the ground. Then switch arms.
- See how many hand taps you can get in 45 seconds.

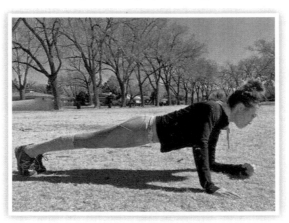

9. One Leg Plank

- This exercise is done just like Plank except one leg is lifted off of the ground as you hold.

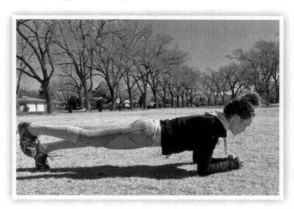

10. 90-Degree Straight Leg Toe Touch

- Lie flat on your back with legs extending straight up at a 90-degree angle.
- Keep your legs straight and your feet right over your hips. Lift your upper body off of the ground and touch your toes.
- Slowly lower back down to the starting position.

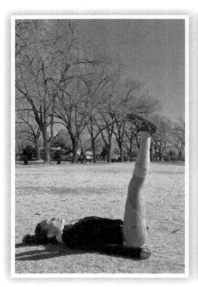
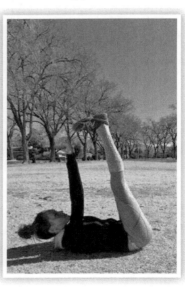

11. Twisted Straight Leg Toe Touch

- This exercise is done just like the 90-Degree Straight Leg Toe Touch (Link to "90-Degree Straight Leg Toe Touch) except you reach for the opposite foot so that you twist to the side.

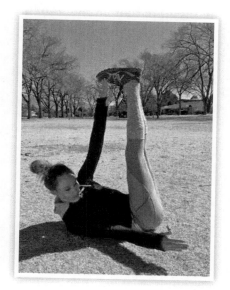

12. Leg Throw Downs

- If you have something stable to hold on to in this pose (like the legs of a heavy chair or the ankles of a friend) use it. Otherwise just keep your arms extended on the ground overhead.
- Lie down flat on your back with legs extending straight up at a 90-degree angle.
- As forcefully as possible (if you have a friend whose ankles you are using ask them to do this) throw your legs down towards the ground, stopping them from hitting the ground by using your core.
- Slowly raise your legs back up to the starting position. This is one rep.

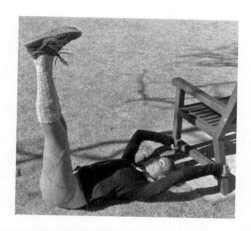

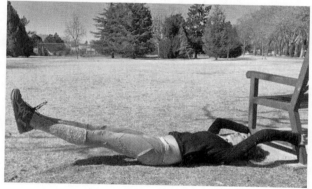

13. Reverse Knee To Nose

- Come onto all fours with straight arms and legs.
- Lift one foot off of the ground, bend the knee, and bring it to your nose. Pause here before kicking the leg out from under you and extending it back.
- Without allowing the foot to touch the ground, immediately do the next rep.

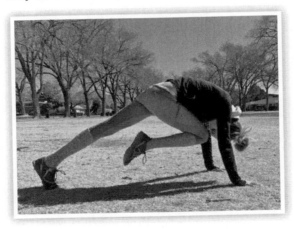

14. Elevators

- Come onto all fours with straight arms and legs.
- Lift one foot off of the ground, bend the knee, and bring it outside the body to the upper arm. Press the knee against the arm and slowly lower it down to the wrist and then back up again.
- Lowering the knee down and back up is one rep.

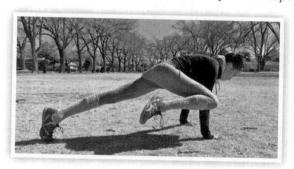

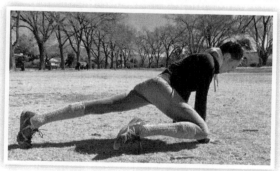

15. Switched Elevators

- This exercise is done just like Elevators only the knee is brought under the body and to the outside of the opposite arm.

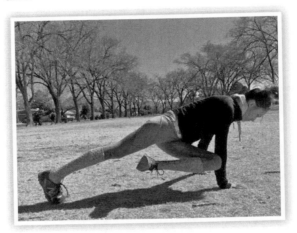

16. Paper Clip

- Lie on your back with legs extending straight up at a 90-degree angle.
- Extend your arms over your head and then lift your upper body off of the ground, reaching for your toes.
- Staying in this crunch position, open your arms and legs out to the side as wide as possible. Bring them back together and then lower the upper body back down to the ground.
- Keep your legs at a 90-degree angle between reps.

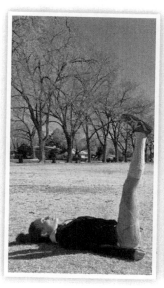
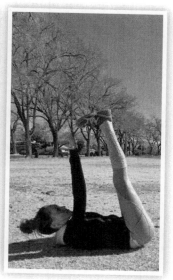

17. Sole Sit Ups

- Lie down on your back and bring the soles of your feet together. Let the knees open and fall to the sides.
- Lift your feet an inch or two off of the ground.
- Bring your hands behind your head with the elbows extended to the sides.
- Keeping the feet lifted, lift your upper body off of the ground to perform a crunch. Lower your body down slowly, but keep your feet off of the ground in between reps.

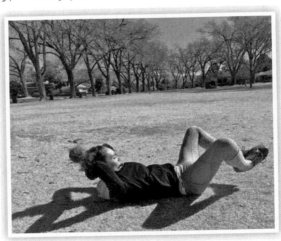

18. Sprinkler Sit Ups

- Lie down on your back with legs extended straight in front of you.
- Extend your arms to the sides of your body, making a "t" shape.
- Use your core to sit up from this position and touch your hand to your opposite foot. Lie back down slowly and then repeat on the other side. This is one rep.

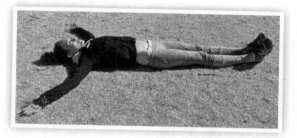

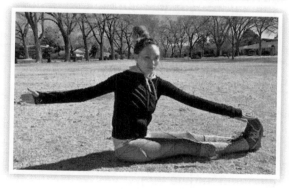

19. Bicycle Crunches

- Lie on your back with knees bent and feet lifted off of the ground.
- Bring your hands behind your head with elbows extending to the sides.
- Keep one leg bent as you straighten the other, hovering it just a few inches above the ground. Simultaneously, bring your opposite elbow to the bent knee. Pause in this position before switching legs and bringing your other elbow across your body to the opposite knee.
- One crunch on each side is one rep.

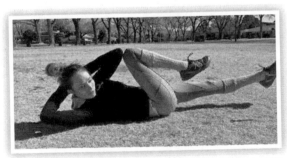

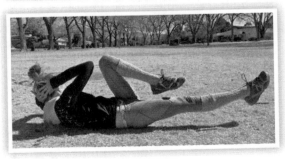

20. Side Forearm Raises

- Come onto your forearms in Plank position.
- Keep your arms just as they are, but take the outside of one foot to the ground and stack the other foot on top.
- Lift the hips up as high as you can and then lower them back down so that they are parallel with the ground.

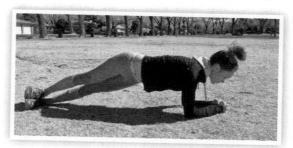

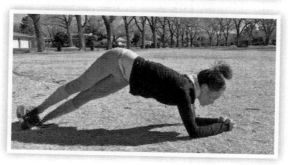

21. Elephant Lift

- Sit on the ground with one leg extended straight in front and the other knee bent.
- Bring your arm under the bent knee and place both hands flat on the ground outside your hips.
- Squeeze your thighs together and use your core to lift your hips, legs, and feet off of the ground. Hold this position for as long as you can, aiming for 15 to 20 seconds on each side -- this is one set.

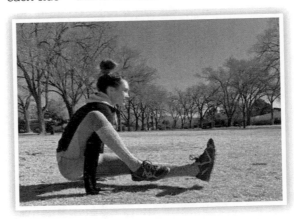

22. Straight Leg Lateral Lifts

- Lie flat on your back with legs lifted at a 90-degree angle.
- Keeping the legs together, lower them to one side as much as possible. Don't let the shoulders come off of the ground. Pause here and then bring the legs back to center.
- Lower your legs to the other side to complete one rep.

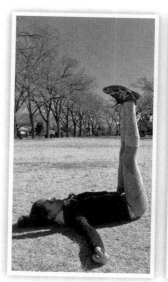 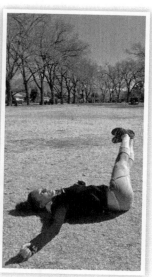

23. Russian Twist

- Lie on your back with knees bent and feet off the ground.
- Do a crunch, bringing your hands together to the outside of your leg.
- Come back to center, lowering your shoulders towards the ground but not allowing them to touch. Reach your arms to the other side to finish one rep.

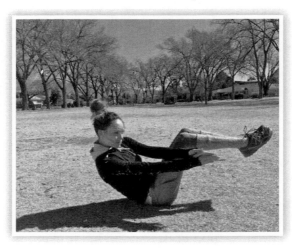

24. Lateral Leg Lift with Toe Touch

- Stand straight with your feet together.
- Lift your leg out to the side, keeping it as straight as possible.
- Reach to the side and try to touch the toes of your lifted leg before coming back to the starting position.
- Do all of your reps on one side before switching legs.

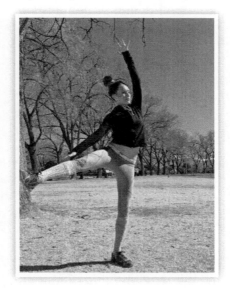

25. Reclined Lateral Toe Touch

- Lie down on your side with your legs stacked on top of each other and feet flexed.
- Lift your top leg up, keeping it as straight as possible, then reach your top hand over to touch your lifted toes. Lower back down to the starting position slowly.
- Do all of your reps on one side before switching legs.

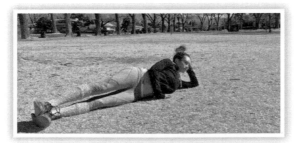

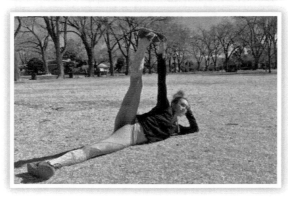

26. Elevated Plank

- This exercise is done just like Plank only the feet are elevated to increase difficulty.

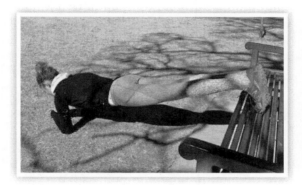

27. Elevated Single Leg Plank

- This exercise is done just like Elevated Plank only one leg is lifted off of the elevated surface.

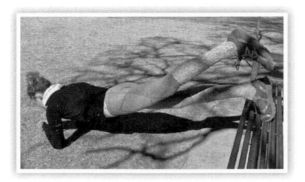

28. Forearm Side Plank with Bottom Leg Lift

- Lie down on your side with legs stacked on top of each other.
- Lift onto your forearm, placing your top hand on your hip.
- Lift the bottom leg off of the ground and bring the knee towards the bottom hand. Slowly return to the starting position.
- Do all of the reps on one side before switching legs.

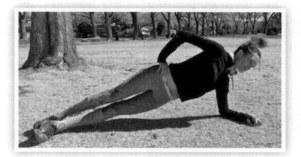

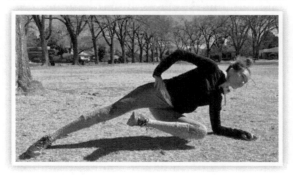

29. Straight Leg Crunches

- Lie down flat on your back with legs at a ninety-degree angle and hands behind your head. Perform crunches like regular, keeping the legs straight.

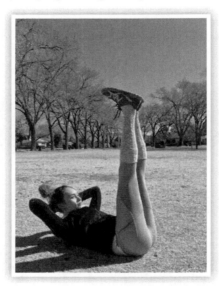

30. Straight Leg Sit Ups

- Lie down flat on your back with legs and arms extended straight.
- Keeping your legs down and without using your hands, sit up and reach for your toes.
- Slowly lower back down to the starting position to complete one rep.

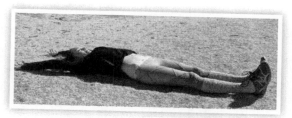

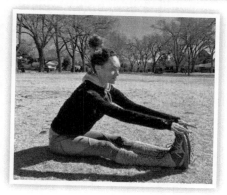

31. Twisted Crunches

- Lie on your back with knees bent and feet flat on the ground.
- Lower your knees to one side, trying to keep them stacked on top of each other.
- Place your hands behind your head with elbows wide. Crunch straight up and then lower slowly back to the ground.
- Do all your reps on one side before switching.

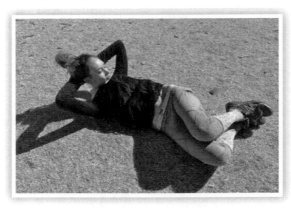

32. Boogie Board Crunches (Boogie Board)

- Lie on your back, bend your knees and lift your feet off the ground.
- Lower your knees to one side, but keep the feet and knees off of the ground.
- Crunch up and reach to the opposite side of your legs.
- Bring your knees to the other side and crunch again to finish one rep.

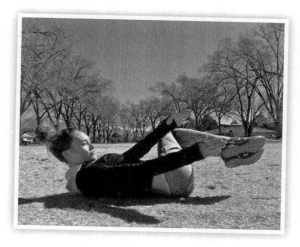

33. Double Crunch

- Lie flat on your back with knees bent.
- Bring your hands behind your head with elbows extended wide.
- Lift your shoulders off the ground to perform a crunch. Hold here in this position before sitting all the way up.
- Lower back down to the ground slowly to finish one rep.

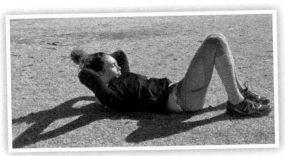

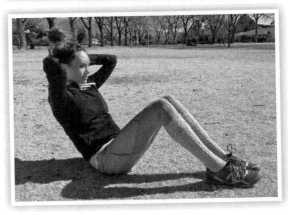

34. Ab Circles

- Sit down on the ground, leaning back to balance on your sit bones. Bring your hands behind your body for extra support.
- Bend your knees and lift your feet off of the ground.
- Make circles with your knees, exaggerating the motion as much as possible. Go slowly!
- One full circle is one rep.
- To make this exercise more difficult, keep the legs straight and make circles with your feet!

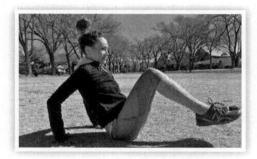

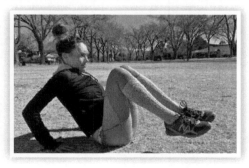

35. Open and Close

- Lie flat on your back with legs extended straight in front of you.
- Keep the legs straight and lift them a few inches off of the ground.
- Move the feet apart and back together to finish one rep.

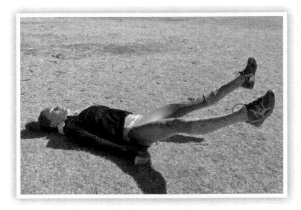

36. IT Crunches

- Lie flat on your back with knees bent and feet flat on the floor.
- Cross one ankle over the other thigh, flexing the foot.
- Bring your hands behind your head with elbows wide.
- Lift your shoulders off of the ground to come into a crunch, bringing your opposite elbow to the knee of the crossed leg.
- Do all of your reps on one side before switching legs.

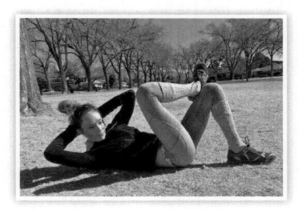

37. Crossed Open and Close

- This exercise is done just like Open and Close but when the feet are brought back together they cross, one leg on top and the other on the bottom.
- Each time after you open your legs to the sides, alternate which leg crosses on top.
- One rep is crossing the left leg on top and then the right.

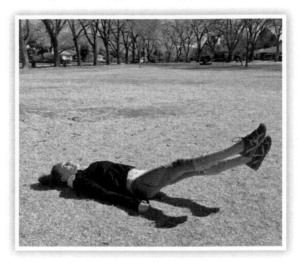

38. Frog Kicks

- Lie on your back with knees bent and feet lifted off of the ground.
- Bend your knees as much as possible, bringing the knees towards your shoulders.
- Kick the feet out in front of you, straightening the legs and pause before bringing them back to the starting position.

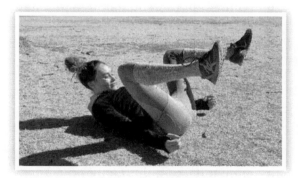

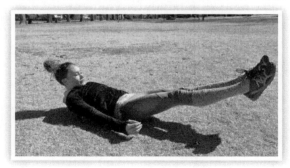

Total Body

1. Walking Planks

   - Come into a Plank position on your forearms.
   - One arm at a time, come off of your forearms and onto your hands. Hold at the top of a push up position for a moment before lowering back down to your forearms. This is one full rep.

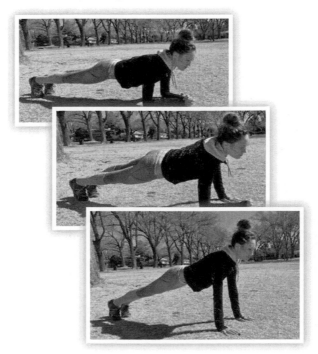

2. Simple Burpees

- Stand with your feet together.
- Bend your knees and bring your hands down to the ground. Plant your hands firmly.
- Hop back into the top of a push up position with arms and legs straight. Hold here for a moment.
- Hop your feet forward in between your hands with bent knees.
- Return to a standing position. This is one rep.

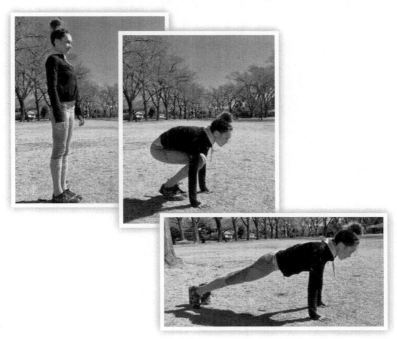

3. Push Up Burpees

- These are done just like the Simple Burpees except instead of just holding the top of push up before jumping forward you actually do a push up.

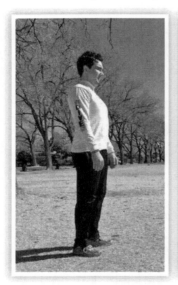
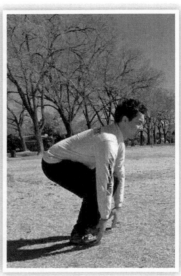

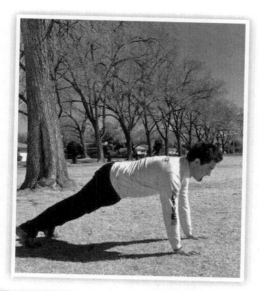

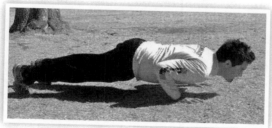

4. Full Side Plank with Leg Lift

- Start in a push up position with arms and legs straight.
- Take the outside of one foot to the ground and stack your other foot on top.
- Balancing on one arm, lift the top leg as high as possible. Pause in this position for a moment before lowering the leg back down.
- Do all of your reps on one side before switching.

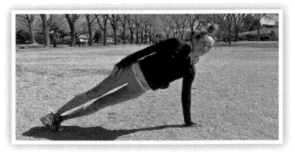

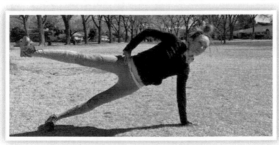

5. Dragon Walks

- Come into the top of a push up with straight arms and legs.
- Lower into a push up while stepping one foot forward, bringing the knee towards the elbow.
- Press back up to the top of a push up and walk your opposite hand forward, stepping that foot forward, knee to elbow.
- Continue moving along the ground in this manner for as long as you can, shooting for 30 seconds. This is one set.

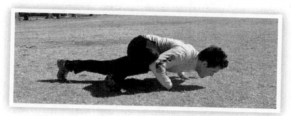

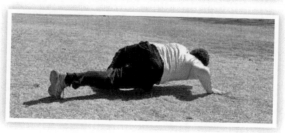

6. Push Up Crawl

- Come into the top of a push up with straight arms and legs.
- Bend the elbows and lower down into the bottom of a push up. Holding this position, crawl along the ground, taking small steps with your hands and feet.
- Continue moving along the ground in this manner for as long as you can, shooting for 30 seconds. This is one set.

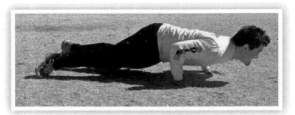

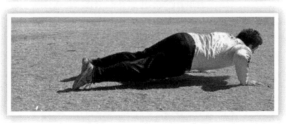

7. Speed Skater

- Stand with feet wide apart and a slight bend in the knees.
- Lift one foot off of the ground and behind you. Lean forward and touch the toes of your front foot with your opposite hand.
- Lower your lifted leg to the ground, stepping wide.
- Then alternate hand and foot, repeating on the other side.

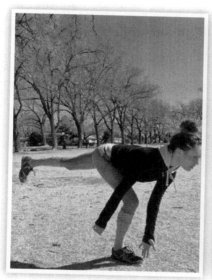 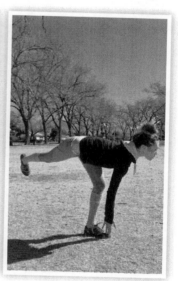

8. Super Speed Skater

- Stand with feet wide apart and a slight bend in the knees.
- Cross one leg behind the other, bending the knees deeper and coming into a lunge-like position.
- Uncross the back leg and hop to the side as wide as you can, landing in the same crossed lunge-like position on the other side. This is one full rep.

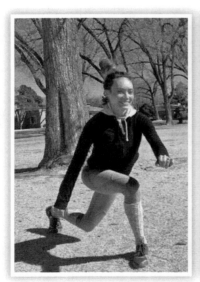
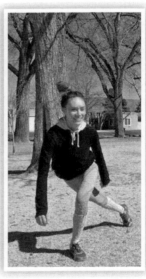

9. Table Top Kicks

- Sit down on the ground and then press yourself up into a table top position – knees bent, ankles under knees, arms straight, hands under shoulders, body parallel to the ground.
- Kick one leg into the air, touching the toes with the opposite hand.
- Come back to the starting position and do the exercise again on the other side. This is one rep.

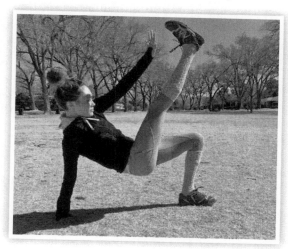

10. Superman

- Lie on your stomach with legs straight and arms extending out in front.
- Lift the arms and the legs off of the ground, keeping the insides of the legs touching.
- Look forward but don't crane the neck up.
- Hold this position for as long as you can, shooting for 30 to 45 seconds. This is one set.

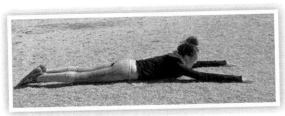

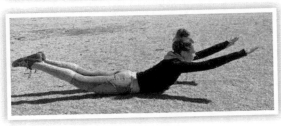

11. One Leg Toe Touch

- Stand tall with straight legs.
- Lift one foot off of the ground and extend the leg out behind you. Start to lower the body down, stopping when you have lowered the body so that it is parallel to the ground. Reach your arms out in front of you. (You should look like a capital letter "T".)
- Hinging from the hips, touch your standing foot and then lift your torso back up so that it is once again in a straight line with your back leg. This is one rep.

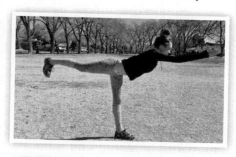

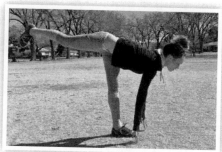

12. One Leg Twisted Toe Touch

- These are done just like the One Leg Toe Touch except instead of reaching down to touch your foot with both hands, reach down with the opposite hand.

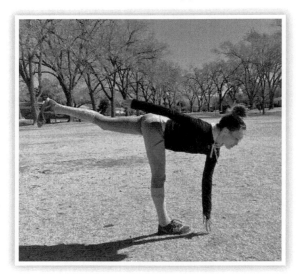

13. Star Jumps

- Stand in an easy squat with knees slightly bent and feet just wider than shoulder-width.
- Explode into a jump, reaching your arms and legs out to the sides and as straight as possible.
- Land back into the starting position with bent knees. This is one rep.

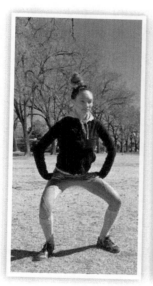
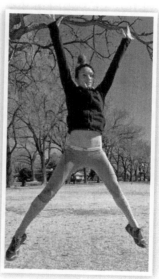

14. Mountain Climbers

- Come to all fours with straight arms and straight legs, like the top of a push up.
- Hop one foot forward towards your hands, bending the knee.
- Hop again to switch feet. This is one rep.

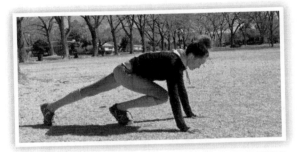

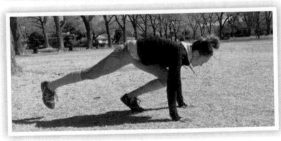

15. Ice Climbers

- These are done just like Mountain Climbers only instead of hopping the foot straight forward, hop it across towards the opposite hand.

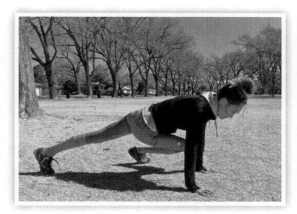

16. Tuck Jumps

- Stand with your feet together, knees slightly bent.
- Explode into a jump, hugging the knees into the chest while in the air.
- Land back in the starting position to finish one rep.

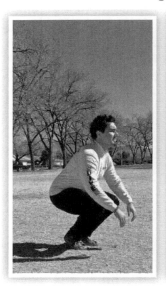
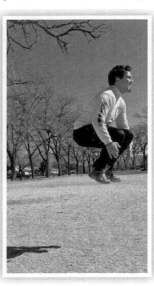

17. Firework Pikes (Firework 1 and 2)

- Come onto all fours with straight arms and bent knees.
- Lift onto the balls of your feet, look forward, and propel your body forward.
- Jump your legs up as high as possible, opening the legs to the sides as you do so.
- The goal is to ultimately get your hips directly over you shoulders with the legs perpendicular to the ground.
- Land back in the starting position to finish one rep.

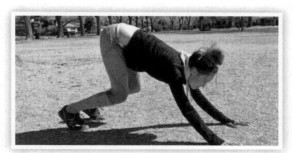

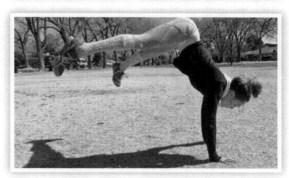

18. Tuck, Roll, Jump

- Lie on your back, hugging your knees in towards your chest.
- Rock back to gain momentum and propel yourself forward to stand.
- Once standing, jump as high as you can. Land with bent knees, immediately coming back to the starting position on your back. This is one rep.

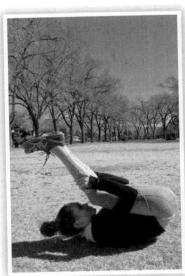
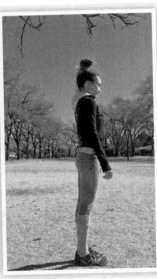

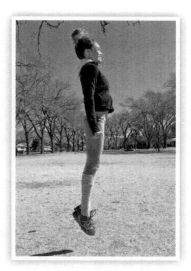

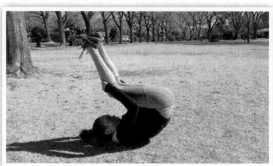

19. Easy Russian Dance

- Sit down and then lift up into a tabletop position – knees bent, feet under knees, arms straight, hands under shoulders, body parallel to the ground.
- Lower your hips slightly towards the ground while kicking one leg out in front of you. At the same time, lift your opposite hand and reach for the toes of the lifted leg. Come back to the starting position before switching sides to complete the rep.

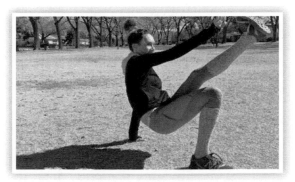

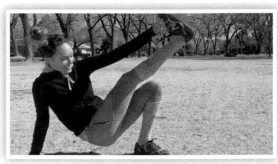

20. Push Up to Side Plank

- Start this exercise by performing a regular Push Up.
- After you have completed one push up, rock to the side and reach your top hand over your head.
- Come back to the top of the push up and repeat the reach on the other side to finish one rep.

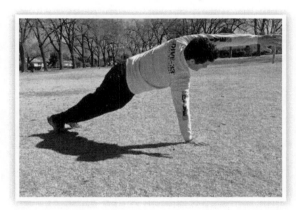

21. Wall Run

- You will need a wall or some sort of sturdy vertical surface to do this exercise.
- Facing away from the wall, come into a push up position with straight arms and legs elevated on the surface, parallel to the ground.
- Take one leg off the wall, bend the knee and bring it towards your shoulder. Place the leg back on the wall and then repeat with the other leg to finish one rep.

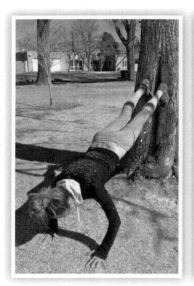 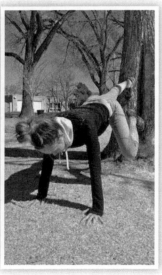

22. Plank Leg Lifts

- Come into a plank position on your forearms with your body parallel to the ground.
- Keeping the legs and body straight, lift one leg up as high as you can.
- Repeat all of the reps on one side before switching legs.

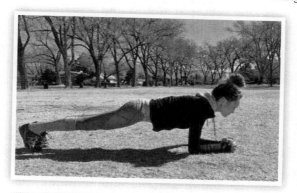

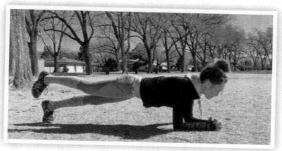

23. Lateral Plank Leg Lifts

- This exercise is done just like Plank Leg Lifts but instead of lifting the leg straight up, extend the leg to the side.
- Keep the body parallel to the ground and the leg as straight as possible.

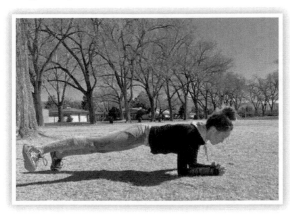

POWER YOGA SESSION

Yoga is a great way to cross-train and give yourself a break from a "regular" workout. No counting reps, just focus on your breath. Work to create fluidity as you move from one pose to the next, moving gracefully and intentionally. Despite the difficulty that can come from some of the poses, yoga is all about finding a balance between effort and ease in everything you do.

The following sequence comes from Julie Schoen's **Flat Tummy Yoga.** It's a great resource for more yoga workouts just like this one that are designed to flatten and tone your tummy!

Power Yoga Benefits: This sequence should be repeated as many times as possible or until you are able to increase your heart rate and work up a bit of a sweat. Burning calories through cardiovascular exercise is one of the keys to getting a flat tummy -- no one can see how strong your stomach is if you have a bit too much around the middle! The goal should be to work your way up to doing 10 to 12 of these flows each day.

As you flow from one pose to the next, remember to keep the core engaged – pulling the navel up and in on folds and then using its strength to transition from one to the next. Use the breath to guide you, moving with each inhalation and exhalation. The goal should be to eventually move quickly through the poses. However, feel free to hold a pose longer if it feels good or if you need a little breather.

1. Tadasana with Anjali Mudra (Mountain Pose with Offering Seal)

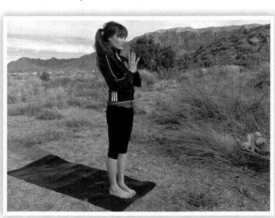

Stand at the top of your mat with your hands in Anjali Mudra (palms pressing together at heart center). Feel your feet ground down, balancing the weight of your body through all four corners. It should feel like you are actually pressing the ground away from you. Lengthen both sides of the ankles and gently engage the muscles of the thighs by lifting the kneecaps. Roll the inner thighs back to help create more space in your lower back. Scoop the tailbone down and under to help the spine curve naturally, protecting the lower back from over arching. Feel the vertebrae of the spine naturally stack on top of each other as you lengthen your back by feeling as if someone is pulling you straight up by a string attached to the top of your head. Keep your chin parallel to the ground and the neck long on all four sides.

As you breathe in this pose, feel free to shut your eyes, working on maintaining your center of gravity. Stay in this pose for as long as you'd like – there's a lot of benefit to learning how to stand properly!

2. Urdhva Hastasana (Upward Salute)

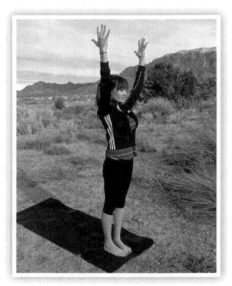

Inhale, bring your hands overhead, keeping the shoulders relaxed and bringing your gaze up. Try to keep the same alignment from Tadasana – it's harder when you extend your arms so really pay attention to your hips and lower back. Allow the chest to open and expand evenly across the collarbones and shoulder blades as you feel a gentle stretch through the shoulders.

3. Uttanasana (Standing Forward Bend Image)

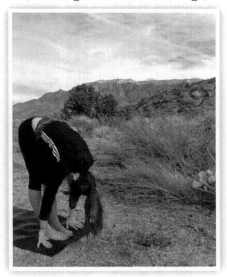

Exhale, bending from the hips, bring the hands down to the ground. If your hands do not touch, allow them to rest on your shins or thighs. Allow the head to be heavy so that your neck can relax and lengthen. Keep the legs strong and engaged by pulling the kneecaps up. To more effectively perform this pose, pull the lower abdomen up and in. The spine should feel like it is lengthening as you continue to get deeper and deeper into the fold.

4. Ardha Uttanasana (Standing Half Forward Bend) -- Ardha Uttanasana Image

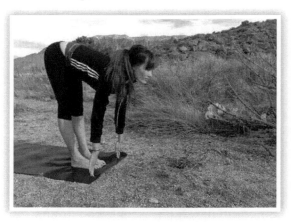

Inhale and bring your hands to your shins. Open the chest forward and gently squeeze the shoulder blades together. Keep your hips directly over the ankles and your gaze forward.

5. Plank Pose -- Plank Image

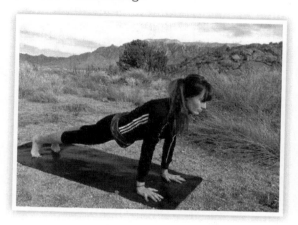

Exhale and hop or step back into Plank Pose, aligning your hands so that they are directly under your shoulders and making sure that your body is parallel with the floor. Engage the core and as you inhale bring your gaze slightly forward.

6. Chaturanga Dandasana (Four-Limbed Staff Pose)

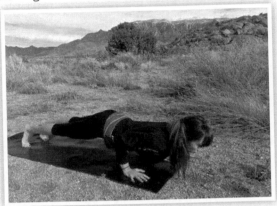

Exhale and lower down to Chaturanga. Keep the body parallel to the mat and the elbows in close to the body. Your elbows should never go above the shoulders in this pose in order to keep the shoulder joint safe. Look forward and keep the neck and spine long. If you need to drop the knees in this pose until you build enough strength feel free to do so.

7. Urdhva Mukha Svanasana (Upward Facing Dog Pose)

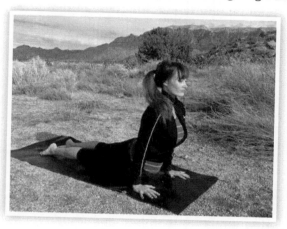

Inhale, press up into Upward Facing Dog by rolling the body forward and lifting the hips and legs off the mat. With your hands directly under the shoulders, push the upper body forward between the arms, opening the chest. If there is too much pressure on the lower back in this pose, you can drop the hips and legs down to the ground and practice Bhujangasana (Cobra Pose) instead.

8. Adho Mukha Svanasana (Downward Facing Dog)

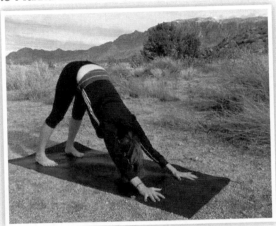

Exhale, bring the hands back over your head and down on the mat in front of you. Spread the fingers wide and press up into Down Dog by straightening the arms and legs. Press the hands into the mat and lift up and out of the shoulders. Your feet should be hip-width apart with the heels directly behind the toes. Engage the legs by lifting the kneecaps and rolling the inner thighs back. Focus on lengthening the back body, especially the spine, with each breath.

To help loosen the neck, feel free to shake your head up and down, yes and no while in this pose.

9. Tri Pada Adho Mukha Svanasana (Three Legged Downward Facing Dog) -- Three Legged Down Dog Image

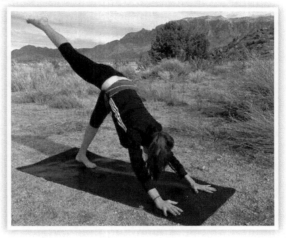

Inhale as you lift one leg up towards the sky, doing your best to keep both hips in one line as you do so. Try to find balance in your body by centering the weight and distributing it evenly between both hands.

10. High Lunge -- High Lunge Image

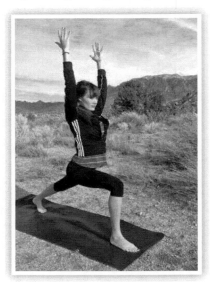

Exhale and step one foot forward between your hands, lifting into High Lunge. The knee of your front leg should be
bent directly over the ankle, making the thigh parallel to the
mat. The back leg should be straight and lifted, balancing on
the ball of the foot. Lift the arms up overhead, but keep the
shoulders and neck relaxed. As you lift your arms, feel your
sides and the space between your ribs lengthen.

Return to Plank and repeat the poses on the other side.

11. Utkatasana (Chair Pose)

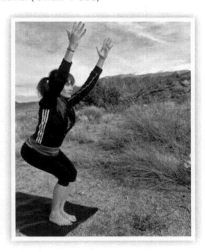

Inhale as you step the back foot forward to meet the front foot. (Alternately, you could step back from High Lunge into Plank and repeat Chaturanga Dandasana, Urdhva Mukha Svanasana, and Adho Mukha Svanasana before coming into this pose.)

With the sides of your feet touching, bend your knees as if you are going to sit down in a chair behind you. Keep the weight in your heels and sit down lower. Raise your arms over your head, making sure that the chest stays lifted and the shoulder joints and neck stay loose and relaxed.

Straighten your legs and return to Tadasana to repeat this sequence.

BALANCE THE BURN – SIMPLE STRETCHES FOR DAILY USE

It's important to stretch every day, especially when working out. Don't rush through the stretches and definitely don't skip them – this is what keeps you and your muscles healthy!

The following stretches are from another book in the **Keep Calm** series, **Keep Calm and Stretch**. It's a great resource to learn more about the importance of stretching, how to maximize its benefits, and other super effective ways to stretch.

1. Elbow Behind Head

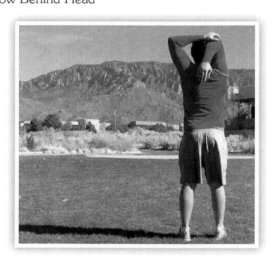

Benefits:

Stretches and increases the range of motion of the shoulders, a common site of stiffness and chronic pain.

How-To:

Standing tall, lift one arm straight into the air with the palm of the hand facing back. Place the hand on your upper back while using the other hand to gently pull your elbow closer towards the center of your head. Find a balance between pressing your elbow down and lifting the elbow up so as to create resistance as you stretch. As your range of motion increases, you can start to move the hand further down your back or try the bound stretch below.

2. Wide Legged Forward Fold (Insert Image 0564)

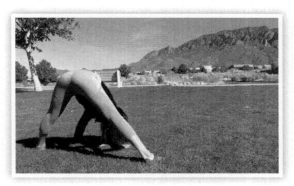

Benefits:

Stretches the hamstrings and inner thighs while lengthening the spine and loosening the muscles of the shoulders and neck. It is also great for relieving stress.

How-To:

Stand with your legs wide apart and feet parallel to each other. Squeeze the shoulder blades together to keep the back straight as you bend forward from the hips. When you have gone as low as you comfortably can, release the neck, shoulders, and back so that they can lengthen and relax. Bring your hands down under the shoulders or grab onto the outsides of your feet. To increase flexibility and strength, keep the fronts of the legs engaged by lifting the kneecaps.

3. Wide Legged Lunge

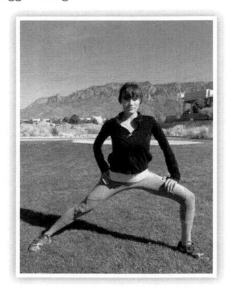

Benefits:

Stretches the inner thigh and groin muscles, helping to prevent injury while relieving tension in the lower back.

How-To:

Stand with your legs wide apart and feet parallel to each other. Bend one knee so that you lower into a side lunge keeping the bent knee right over the ankle. For a deeper stretch increase the distance between your feet.

4. Gorilla Stretch

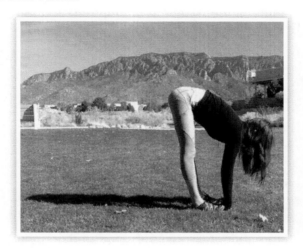

Benefits:

Stretches the entire back body, especially the backs of the legs and the area between the shoulder blades, and relieves the wrists and fingers of discomfort.

How-To:

Stand with your feet hip-width apart. Fold forward, bending the knees if necessary, to bring your hands to your feet. Slide your hands palms up under the soles of your feet so that your toes are touching the crease of your wrist. Rock forward to bring more weight into the ball of your foot providing a better stretch for your upper back and wrists. If you are barefoot, you can move the toes up and down to massage the wrists.

5. Standing Shoulder Twist

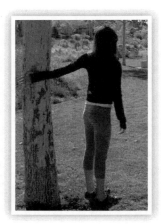

Benefits:

Stretches deep into the muscles of the shoulders and upper back. Because of the tendency to slouch forward throughout the day, this pose is essential in order to strengthen and loosen the muscles of the upper back and shoulders while improving posture. For this stretch you will need some sort of sturdy vertical object, such as a wall, tree, pole, or even another person.

How-To:

Stand close enough to a vertical surface so that one side of your body is either flush to it (like if you are using a wall) or so that your feet are in line with it and a foot or so in front. Extend your arm back so that the palm of your hand can touch the surface, thumb on top. Deepen the stretch by pressing your hand into the surface as you twist away from it.

6. Heel To Butt Stretch (Insert Image 0652)

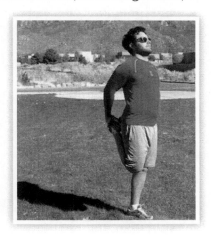

Benefits:

Stretches the front of the upper leg and hip flexor while improving balance, which is good for the brain and great for injury prevention.

How-To:

It is a good idea to start using a wall or tree for balance but you can do this pose without as well.

Stand tall with your feet together. Lift one foot off the ground, bending the knee and bringing your heel to your butt. Keep both knees together as much as possible. To increase the stretch pull the foot closer to your butt with your hands while you simultaneously kick the foot back into your hand.

7. Standing Calf Stretch

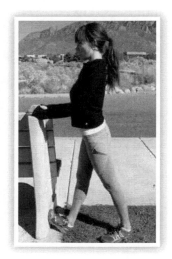

Benefits:

This pose is very straightforward, but it is one of the best ways to, as the name implies, stretch the calf muscle at the back of your leg.

How-To:

Find a surface that you can press your foot into, such as a wall, a tree, or a curb.

Stand so that you can place the sole of the foot onto the surface while keeping the heel on the ground. Intensify the stretch by pressing your foot firmly against the surface and placing more of the sole of your foot onto the surface.

8. Arm Across Chest

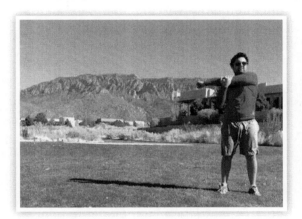

Benefits:

Uses resistance to stretch and increase the flexibility of the upper arm and shoulder.

How-To:

Bring one arm across the body at shoulder height with the elbow slightly bent. Use your other hand to press the upper arm in towards your chest. Simultaneously, draw the shoulder of the arm that is being stretched back into its socket. The resistance created by doing this will help to increase the flexibility of your shoulder faster than just simply pressing the arm into the chest.

9. Knee Down Lunge

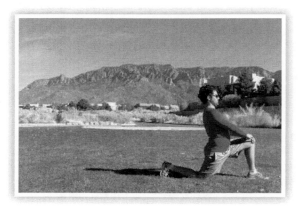

Benefits:

Refines balance while stretching and strengthening the muscles surrounding the hips.

How-To:

Stand tall with your feet hip width apart. Take a big step forward with one of your feet and bring the knee of the back leg down to the ground. Adjust your stance so that you feel a stretch in the hip of the back leg and so that the knee of your front leg is directly over the ankle. Press back into the foot of the back leg as you simultaneously lower your hips down closer to the ground.

10. Runner's Lunge (Insert Image 0645)

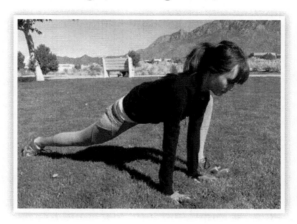

Benefits:

This stretch works on improving the flexibility of the hips, hamstrings, and thighs.

How-To:

Come down to all fours. Extend one leg straight back behind you, keeping the knee lifted of the ground and weight in the ball of the foot. Step the front foot forward so that it is even with your hands. Both hands should be placed on the inside of the front foot. Press the hips down and keep the back straight. To create resistance, continue pressing back through the extended back leg and into the ball of the foot.

11. Easy Seated Twist

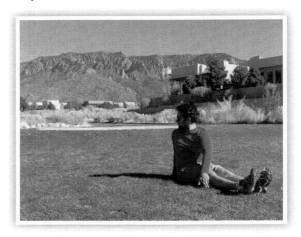

Benefits:

Gently stretches the back, helping to increase flexibility and decrease discomfort created from sitting for long periods of time.

How-To:

Sit on the ground with your legs extended straight out in front of you. Keep the legs together as you bring the left hand to the outside of the right leg. Place your right hand on the ground at the base of spine to help you twist further while maintaining a long spine. As you inhale, use the right hand to sit up straighter. As you exhale, use the left hand to help you twist around further.

12. Seated Forward Fold

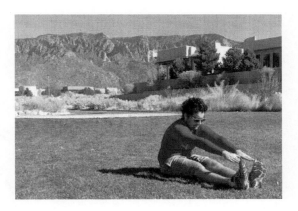

Benefits:

This stretch helps to calm and soothe the mind while lowering blood pressure and providing an intense opening for the entire back of the body.

How-To:

Sit on the ground with legs extended straight out in front of you. Flex the feet back towards the face and press the thighbones firmly down into the ground. Sit up as tall as possible and squeeze the shoulder blades together slightly to help keep the back straight and engaged. Keeping a straight spine, start to slowly fold forward from the hips, reaching for your toes. The stretch comes from folding at the hip crease and flexing the legs, not from getting as low as possible.

13. Supine One Leg Pull (Insert Image 0633)

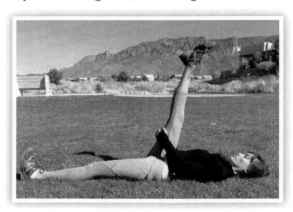

Benefits:

Increases flexibility of the hips while stretching the back of the lifted leg.

How-To:

Lie down flat on your back with your legs extended straight in front of you. Begin to lift one of your legs into the air. Try to keep both legs straight and the bottom leg on the ground. Grab onto the back of the thigh of the lifted leg and gently pull it closer towards your body. If you cannot keep the shoulders on the ground, use something like a dog leash around the lifted leg so that you can pull on the leash to bring your leg closer while keeping your spine flat along the ground. To create resistance in this stretch, use your arms to pull your leg in as your leg pushes away from your body.

And Don't Miss Out On The Rest Of The
Keep Calm Series!

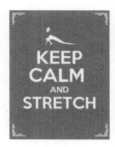   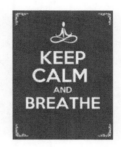

Keep Calm and Stretch   Keep Calm and Breathe

Discover All of **Little Pearl's** Awesome Books!
(http://www.amazon.com/Little-Pearl/e/B007UKU5D0/)

and learn more about Yoga Instructor and
author **Julie Schoen**
(http://www.amazon.com/Julie-Schoen/e/B007GA0A3E/)

Little Pearl Would also like to introduce you to our friends
at **Silver Bullet Books**
(http://www.amazon.com/Silver-Bullet/e/B00B10N6HM/)

Printed in Great Britain
by Amazon.co.uk, Ltd.,
Marston Gate.